First Things First

Why keep a health diary???

This is a great question and the answer is great as well. In fact I am going to give you 5 great answers …

1. You can't change what you don't know …

Sometimes you can't sleep at night? Or maybe you keep getting a skin rash or you feel very lethargic at times? If you suffer minor health issues but are not sure why they appear, keeping a health diary of your exercise regime and your food and fluid intake can help you identify patterns that may be causing you health problems.

2. Keep from falling into a rut …

Your diary will help warn you when you are going off track. Binging on the sweet stuff, too much coffee, or too few rest days between your heavy exercise regime causing health problems? Journalling will help you notice a trend.

3. Easier to stay on track …

Keeping a diary holds you accountable, especially important if you are doing this health journey solo. By recording in your health diary everyday you are making a conscious decision to stick to your health plan. Even if some days aren't always healthy days, at least you will know it and can compensate for it.

4. Record how lifestyle choices influence your food intake and vice versa …

Lifestyle choices play a role in what you eat and how much you eat. Diet plays a massive role in your physical and mental health. By tracking your lifestyle and diet choices you will be better able to understand and change the relationship between these two important factors and your overall health.

5. It is really motivating …

I fill in my diary everyday and I love it when I can see that I am sticking to my exercise routine and my diet plan. I find this process really motivating and it challenges me to continue to do better.

"If you lack direction in your life and feel you have achieved nothing keep a diary. A diary will show you in which direction you are heading and how many great goals you achieve everyday of your life." – Jennifer Daniels

Heathy Food Alternatives

Breakfast Ideas

1. Whey Protein – if you are into protein drinks then whey is a great way to start your day. Whey powers your muscles so blend some with milk or water.
2. Porridge – as long as you cook your own oats. Oats are crammed with vitamin B and iron, and they're filling. Instead of sugar, add diced fresh fruit or natural yoghurt.
3. Eggs – the cholesterol is good for building your muscles and you can add any variety of fresh, lightly saute'ed vegetables.
4. Toast – according to research done by Lund University white rye bread is the best and you can make it even better by spreading avocado on it rather then butter or magarine.
5. Green Tea – instead of coffee or normal tea. Green tea is packed full of antioxidants, not caffeine, and it can also accelerate your metabolic rate, so there's no argument, drink green tea.

Lunch Ideas

1. Salads – green , Mediterranean, caesar, tuna, bean, etc., they are all pretty good for you. The main thing to watch out for is the dressing. If you absolutely need it try a sprinkling of olive oil or low fat dressings. But use dressings sparingly.
2. Grilled Chicken – done on a sandwich with some greenery and pineapple pieces is delicious.
3. Wraps – with roast beef, horseradish, lettuce and tomatoes, and a sprinkling of grated cheese on top, is filling and tastes great.
4. Sandwich – turkey and cucumber on white rye bread is a great combination and low calories too. Add a bit of garlic and relish to give the taste an extra hit.
5. Water – it's filling and so damn good for you.

Dinner Ideas (these recipes are online at http://www.jamieoliver.com/recipes)

1. Easy Spelt Pizza
2. Pasta with Aubergine & Tomato Sauce
3. Pork, Spring Green & Black Bean Stir Fry
4. Mexican Chicken Chilli
5. LA Style Turkey Salad
6. Easy Curried Fish Stew
7. Sizzling Steak Stir Fry

Snack Ideas

Instead of chocolate and chips try:
fresh fruit, celery & carrot sticks, nuts, legumes, seeds, beans, raisins, sultanas, dates, natural yoghurt, cottage cheese, hummus …

WEEK ONE: _____

MONDAY

CARDIO:_____
_____
_____

STRENGTH:_____
_____
_____

STRETCHING:_____
_____
_____

DIET:_____
_____
_____

TUESDAY

CARDIO:_____
_____
_____

STRENGTH:_____
_____
_____

STRETCHING:_____
_____
_____

DIET:_____
_____
_____

WEDNESDAY

CARDIO:_____
_____
_____

STRENGTH:_____
_____
_____

STRETCHING:_____

_____

_____

DIET:_____

_____

_____

_____

THURSDAY

CARDIO:_____

_____

_____

STRENGTH:_____

_____

_____

STRETCHING:_____

_____

_____

DIET:_____

_____

_____

FRIDAY

CARDIO:_____

_____

_____

STRENGTH:_____

_____

_____

STRETCHING:_____

_____

_____

DIET:_____

_____

_____

SATURDAY

CARDIO:_____
_____
_____

STRENGTH:_____
_____
_____

STRETCHING:_____
_____
_____

DIET:_____
_____
_____

SUNDAY

CARDIO:_____
_____
_____

STRENGTH:_____
_____
_____

STRETCHING:_____
_____
_____

DIET:_____
_____
_____

WEEKLY NOTES:
_____
_____
_____
_____
_____
_____

"Make time for your health or your health will take time away from you."
– Bruce Taplin (A try hard healthy lifestyle fan)

WEEK TWO: _____

MONDAY

CARDIO:_____

_____

_____

STRENGTH:_____

_____

_____

STRETCHING:_____

_____

_____

DIET:_____

_____

_____

TUESDAY

CARDIO:_____

_____

_____

STRENGTH:_____

_____

_____

STRETCHING:_____

_____

_____

DIET:_____

_____

_____

WEDNESDAY

CARDIO:_____

_____

_____

STRENGTH:_____

_____

_____

STRETCHING:_____

_____

_____

DIET:_____

_____

_____

_____

THURSDAY

CARDIO:_____

_____

_____

STRENGTH:_____

_____

_____

STRETCHING:_____

_____

_____

DIET:_____

_____

_____

FRIDAY

CARDIO:_____

_____

_____

STRENGTH:_____

_____

_____

STRETCHING:_____

_____

_____

DIET:_____

_____

_____

SATURDAY

CARDIO:_____
_____
_____

STRENGTH:_____
_____
_____

STRETCHING:_____
_____
_____

DIET:_____
_____
_____

SUNDAY

CARDIO:_____
_____
_____

STRENGTH:_____
_____
_____

STRETCHING:_____
_____
_____

DIET:_____
_____
_____

WEEKLY NOTES:
_____
_____
_____
_____
_____
_____

"The first wealth is health." – Ralph Waldo Emerson

WEEK THREE: _____

MONDAY

CARDIO:_____
_____
_____

STRENGTH:_____
_____
_____

STRETCHING:_____
_____
_____

DIET:_____
_____
_____

TUESDAY

CARDIO:_____
_____
_____

STRENGTH:_____
_____
_____

STRETCHING:_____
_____
_____

DIET:_____
_____
_____

WEDNESDAY

CARDIO:_____
_____
_____

STRENGTH:_____
_____
_____

STRETCHING:_____

_____

_____

DIET:_____

_____

_____

_____

THURSDAY

CARDIO:_____

_____

_____

STRENGTH:_____

_____

_____

STRETCHING:_____

_____

_____

DIET:_____

_____

_____

FRIDAY

CARDIO:_____

_____

_____

STRENGTH:_____

_____

_____

STRETCHING:_____

_____

_____

DIET:_____

_____

_____

SATURDAY

CARDIO:_____
_____
_____

STRENGTH:_____
_____
_____

STRETCHING:_____
_____
_____

DIET:_____
_____
_____

SUNDAY

CARDIO:_____
_____
_____

STRENGTH:_____
_____
_____

STRETCHING:_____
_____
_____

DIET:_____
_____
_____

WEEKLY NOTES:
_____
_____
_____
_____
_____
_____

"Looking after my health today gives me a better hope for tomorrow" – Anne Wilson Schaef

WEEK FOUR: _____

MONDAY

CARDIO:_____
_____
_____

STRENGTH:_____
_____
_____

STRETCHING:_____
_____
_____

DIET:_____
_____
_____

TUESDAY

CARDIO:_____
_____
_____

STRENGTH:_____
_____
_____

STRETCHING:_____
_____
_____

DIET:_____
_____
_____

WEDNESDAY

CARDIO:_____
_____
_____

STRENGTH:_____
_____
_____

STRETCHING:_____

_____

_____

DIET:_____

_____

_____

_____

THURSDAY

CARDIO:_____

_____

_____

STRENGTH:_____

_____

_____

STRETCHING:_____

_____

_____

DIET:_____

_____

_____

FRIDAY

CARDIO:_____

_____

_____

STRENGTH:_____

_____

_____

STRETCHING:_____

_____

_____

DIET:_____

_____

_____

SATURDAY

CARDIO:_____
_____
_____

STRENGTH:_____
_____
_____

STRETCHING:_____
_____
_____

DIET:_____
_____
_____

SUNDAY

CARDIO:_____
_____
_____

STRENGTH:_____
_____
_____

STRETCHING:_____
_____
_____

DIET:_____
_____
_____

WEEKLY NOTES:
_____
_____
_____
_____
_____
_____

"Health is like money, we never have a true idea of its value until we lose it."
- Josh Billings

WEEK FIVE: _____

MONDAY

CARDIO:_____
_____
_____

STRENGTH:_____
_____
_____

STRETCHING:_____
_____
_____

DIET:_____
_____
_____

TUESDAY

CARDIO:_____
_____
_____

STRENGTH:_____
_____
_____

STRETCHING:_____
_____
_____

DIET:_____
_____
_____

WEDNESDAY

CARDIO:_____
_____
_____

STRENGTH:_____
_____
_____

STRETCHING:_____
_____
_____

DIET:_____
_____
_____
_____

THURSDAY

CARDIO:_____
_____
_____

STRENGTH:_____
_____
_____

STRETCHING:_____
_____
_____

DIET:_____
_____
_____

FRIDAY

CARDIO:_____
_____
_____

STRENGTH:_____
_____
_____

STRETCHING:_____
_____
_____

DIET:_____
_____
_____

SATURDAY

CARDIO:_____
_____
_____

STRENGTH:_____
_____
_____

STRETCHING:_____
_____
_____

DIET:_____
_____
_____

SUNDAY

CARDIO:_____
_____
_____

STRENGTH:_____
_____
_____

STRETCHING:_____
_____
_____

DIET:_____
_____
_____

WEEKLY NOTES:
_____
_____
_____
_____
_____
_____

"Take care of your body. It's the only place you have to live." - *Jim Rohn*

WEEK SIX: _____

MONDAY

CARDIO:_____
_____
_____

STRENGTH:_____
_____
_____

STRETCHING:_____
_____
_____

DIET:_____
_____
_____

TUESDAY

CARDIO:_____
_____
_____

STRENGTH:_____
_____
_____

STRETCHING:_____
_____
_____

DIET:_____
_____
_____

WEDNESDAY

CARDIO:_____
_____
_____

STRENGTH:_____
_____
_____

STRETCHING:_____

_____

_____

DIET:_____

_____

_____

_____

THURSDAY

CARDIO:_____

_____

_____

STRENGTH:_____

_____

_____

STRETCHING:_____

_____

_____

DIET:_____

_____

_____

FRIDAY

CARDIO:_____

_____

_____

STRENGTH:_____

_____

_____

STRETCHING:_____

_____

_____

DIET:_____

_____

_____

SATURDAY

CARDIO:_____
_____
_____

STRENGTH:_____
_____
_____

STRETCHING:_____
_____
_____

DIET:_____
_____
_____

SUNDAY

CARDIO:_____
_____
_____

STRENGTH:_____
_____
_____

STRETCHING:_____
_____
_____

DIET:_____
_____

WEEKLY NOTES:
_____
_____
_____
_____
_____
_____

"Our bodies are our gardens – our wills are our gardeners." - William Shakespeare

WEEK SEVEN: _____

MONDAY

CARDIO:_____
_____
_____

STRENGTH:_____
_____
_____

STRETCHING:_____
_____
_____

DIET:_____
_____
_____

TUESDAY

CARDIO:_____
_____
_____

STRENGTH:_____
_____
_____

STRETCHING:_____
_____
_____

DIET:_____
_____
_____

WEDNESDAY

CARDIO:_____
_____
_____

STRENGTH:_____
_____
_____

STRETCHING:_____

_____

_____

DIET:_____

_____

_____

_____

THURSDAY

CARDIO:_____

_____

_____

STRENGTH:_____

_____

_____

STRETCHING:_____

_____

_____

DIET:_____

_____

_____

FRIDAY

CARDIO:_____

_____

_____

STRENGTH:_____

_____

_____

STRETCHING:_____

_____

_____

DIET:_____

_____

_____

SATURDAY

CARDIO:_____
_____
_____

STRENGTH:_____
_____
_____

STRETCHING:_____
_____
_____

DIET:_____
_____
_____

SUNDAY

CARDIO:_____
_____
_____

STRENGTH:_____
_____
_____

STRETCHING:_____
_____
_____

DIET:_____
_____
_____

WEEKLY NOTES:
_____
_____
_____
_____
_____
_____

"Health is a relationship between you and your body" - *Terri Guillemets*

WEEK EIGHT: _____

MONDAY

CARDIO:_____
_____
_____

STRENGTH:_____
_____
_____

STRETCHING:_____
_____
_____

DIET:_____
_____
_____

TUESDAY

CARDIO:_____
_____
_____

STRENGTH:_____
_____
_____

STRETCHING:_____
_____
_____

DIET:_____
_____
_____

WEDNESDAY

CARDIO:_____
_____
_____

STRENGTH:_____
_____
_____

STRETCHING:_____

_____

_____

DIET:_____

_____

_____

_____

THURSDAY

CARDIO:_____

_____

_____

STRENGTH:_____

_____

_____

STRETCHING:_____

_____

_____

DIET:_____

_____

_____

FRIDAY

CARDIO:_____

_____

_____

STRENGTH:_____

_____

_____

STRETCHING:_____

_____

_____

DIET:_____

_____

_____

SATURDAY

CARDIO:_____
_____
_____

STRENGTH:_____
_____
_____

STRETCHING:_____
_____
_____

DIET:_____
_____
_____

SUNDAY

CARDIO:_____
_____
_____

STRENGTH:_____
_____
_____

STRETCHING:_____
_____
_____

DIET:_____
_____
_____

WEEKLY NOTES:
_____
_____
_____
_____
_____
_____
_____

"They who take medicine and neglect to diet wastes the skill of their doctors."
- Chinese Proverb

WEEK NINE: _____

MONDAY

CARDIO:_____
_____
_____

STRENGTH:_____
_____
_____

STRETCHING:_____
_____
_____

DIET:_____
_____
_____

TUESDAY

CARDIO:_____
_____
_____

STRENGTH:_____
_____
_____

STRETCHING:_____
_____
_____

DIET:_____
_____
_____

WEDNESDAY

CARDIO:_____
_____
_____

STRENGTH:_____
_____
_____

STRETCHING:_____
_____
_____

DIET:_____
_____
_____
_____

THURSDAY

CARDIO:_____
_____
_____

STRENGTH:_____
_____
_____

STRETCHING:_____
_____
_____

DIET:_____
_____
_____

FRIDAY

CARDIO:_____
_____
_____

STRENGTH:_____
_____
_____

STRETCHING:_____
_____
_____

DIET:_____
_____
_____

SATURDAY

CARDIO:_____
_____
_____

STRENGTH:_____
_____
_____

STRETCHING:_____
_____
_____

DIET:_____
_____
_____

SUNDAY

CARDIO:_____
_____
_____

STRENGTH:_____
_____
_____

STRETCHING:_____
_____
_____

DIET:_____
_____

WEEKLY NOTES:
_____
_____
_____
_____
_____
_____

"A man too busy to take care of his health is like a mechanic too busy to take care of his tools." - Spanish Proverb

WEEK TEN: _____

MONDAY

CARDIO:_____
_____
_____

STRENGTH:_____
_____
_____

STRETCHING:_____
_____
_____

DIET:_____
_____
_____

TUESDAY

CARDIO:_____
_____
_____

STRENGTH:_____
_____
_____

STRETCHING:_____
_____
_____

DIET:_____
_____
_____

WEDNESDAY

CARDIO:_____
_____
_____

STRENGTH:_____
_____
_____

STRETCHING:_____

_____

_____

DIET:_____

_____

_____

_____

THURSDAY

CARDIO:_____

_____

_____

STRENGTH:_____

_____

_____

STRETCHING:_____

_____

_____

DIET:_____

_____

_____

FRIDAY

CARDIO:_____

_____

_____

STRENGTH:_____

_____

_____

STRETCHING:_____

_____

_____

DIET:_____

_____

_____

SATURDAY

CARDIO:_____
_____
_____

STRENGTH:_____
_____
_____

STRETCHING:_____
_____
_____

DIET:_____
_____
_____

SUNDAY

CARDIO:_____
_____
_____

STRENGTH:_____
_____
_____

STRETCHING:_____
_____
_____

DIET:_____
_____
_____

WEEKLY NOTES:
_____
_____
_____
_____
_____
_____
_____

"True healthcare reform starts in your kitchen, not in Washington"
- Anonymous

WEEK ELEVEN: _____

MONDAY

CARDIO:_____
_____
_____

STRENGTH:_____
_____
_____

STRETCHING:_____
_____
_____

DIET:_____
_____
_____

TUESDAY

CARDIO:_____
_____
_____

STRENGTH:_____
_____
_____

STRETCHING:_____
_____
_____

DIET:_____
_____
_____

WEDNESDAY

CARDIO:_____
_____
_____

STRENGTH:_____
_____
_____

STRETCHING:_____
_____
_____

DIET:_____
_____
_____
_____

THURSDAY

CARDIO:_____
_____
_____

STRENGTH:_____
_____
_____

STRETCHING:_____
_____
_____

DIET:_____
_____
_____

FRIDAY

CARDIO:_____
_____
_____

STRENGTH:_____
_____
_____

STRETCHING:_____
_____
_____

DIET:_____
_____
_____

SATURDAY

CARDIO:_____
_____
_____

STRENGTH:_____
_____
_____

STRETCHING:_____
_____
_____

DIET:_____
_____
_____

SUNDAY

CARDIO:_____
_____
_____

STRENGTH:_____
_____
_____

STRETCHING:_____
_____
_____

DIET:_____
_____
_____

WEEKLY NOTES:
_____
_____
_____
_____
_____
_____

"To insure good health: eat lightly, breathe deeply, live moderately, cultivate cheerfulness, and maintain an interest in life." - William Londen

WEEK TWELVE: _____

MONDAY

CARDIO:_____
_____
_____

STRENGTH:_____
_____
_____

STRETCHING:_____
_____
_____

DIET:_____
_____
_____

TUESDAY

CARDIO:_____
_____
_____

STRENGTH:_____
_____
_____

STRETCHING:_____
_____
_____

DIET:_____
_____
_____

WEDNESDAY

CARDIO:_____
_____
_____

STRENGTH:_____
_____
_____

STRETCHING:_____

_____

_____

DIET:_____

_____

_____

_____

THURSDAY

CARDIO:_____

_____

_____

STRENGTH:_____

_____

_____

STRETCHING:_____

_____

_____

DIET:_____

_____

_____

FRIDAY

CARDIO:_____

_____

_____

STRENGTH:_____

_____

_____

STRETCHING:_____

_____

_____

DIET:_____

_____

_____

SATURDAY

CARDIO:_____

_____

_____

STRENGTH:_____

_____

_____

STRETCHING:_____

_____

_____

DIET:_____

_____

_____

SUNDAY

CARDIO:_____

_____

_____

STRENGTH:_____

_____

_____

STRETCHING:_____

_____

_____

DIET:_____

_____

_____

WEEKLY NOTES:

_____

_____

_____

_____

_____

_____

"Physical fitness is not only one of the most important keys to a healthy body, it is the basis of dynamic and creative intellectual activity." - John F. Kennedy

WEEK THIRTEEN: _____

MONDAY

CARDIO:_____
_____
_____

STRENGTH:_____
_____
_____

STRETCHING:_____
_____
_____

DIET:_____
_____
_____

TUESDAY

CARDIO:_____
_____
_____

STRENGTH:_____
_____
_____

STRETCHING:_____
_____
_____

DIET:_____
_____
_____

WEDNESDAY

CARDIO:_____
_____
_____

STRENGTH:_____
_____

STRETCHING:_____
_____
_____

DIET:_____
_____
_____
_____

THURSDAY

CARDIO:_____
_____
_____

STRENGTH:_____
_____
_____

STRETCHING:_____
_____
_____

DIET:_____
_____
_____

FRIDAY

CARDIO:_____
_____
_____

STRENGTH:_____
_____
_____

STRETCHING:_____
_____
_____

DIET:_____
_____
_____

SATURDAY

CARDIO:_____
_____
_____

STRENGTH:_____
_____
_____

STRETCHING:_____
_____
_____

DIET:_____
_____
_____

SUNDAY

CARDIO:_____
_____
_____

STRENGTH:_____
_____
_____

STRETCHING:_____
_____
_____

DIET:_____
_____
_____

WEEKLY NOTES:
_____
_____
_____
_____
_____
_____

"If you hate starting over stop quitting!" - *Anonymous*

WEEK FOURTEEN: _____

MONDAY

CARDIO:_____
_____
_____

STRENGTH:_____
_____
_____

STRETCHING:_____
_____
_____

DIET:_____
_____
_____

TUESDAY

CARDIO:_____
_____
_____

STRENGTH:_____
_____
_____

STRETCHING:_____
_____
_____

DIET:_____
_____
_____

WEDNESDAY

CARDIO:_____
_____
_____

STRENGTH:_____
_____
_____

STRETCHING:_____
_____
_____

DIET:_____
_____
_____

THURSDAY

CARDIO:_____
_____
_____

STRENGTH:_____
_____
_____

STRETCHING:_____
_____
_____

DIET:_____
_____
_____

FRIDAY

CARDIO:_____
_____
_____

STRENGTH:_____
_____
_____

STRETCHING:_____
_____
_____

DIET:_____
_____
_____

SATURDAY

CARDIO:_____
_____
_____

STRENGTH:_____
_____
_____

STRETCHING:_____
_____
_____

DIET:_____
_____
_____

SUNDAY

CARDIO:_____
_____
_____

STRENGTH:_____
_____
_____

STRETCHING:_____
_____
_____

DIET:_____
_____
_____

WEEKLY NOTES:
_____
_____
_____
_____
_____
_____
_____

"Your only limit is you." - Anonymous

WEEK FIFTEEN: _____

MONDAY

CARDIO:_____
_____
_____

STRENGTH:_____
_____
_____

STRETCHING:_____
_____
_____

DIET:_____
_____
_____

TUESDAY

CARDIO:_____
_____
_____

STRENGTH:_____
_____
_____

STRETCHING:_____
_____
_____

DIET:_____
_____

WEDNESDAY

CARDIO:_____
_____
_____

STRENGTH:_____
_____
_____

STRETCHING:_____
_____
_____

DIET:_____
_____
_____
_____

THURSDAY

CARDIO:_____
_____
_____

STRENGTH:_____
_____
_____

STRETCHING:_____
_____
_____

DIET:_____
_____
_____

FRIDAY

CARDIO:_____
_____
_____

STRENGTH:_____
_____
_____

STRETCHING:_____
_____
_____

DIET:_____
_____
_____

SATURDAY

CARDIO:_____
_____
_____

STRENGTH:_____
_____
_____

STRETCHING:_____
_____
_____

DIET:_____
_____
_____

SUNDAY

CARDIO:_____
_____
_____

STRENGTH:_____
_____
_____

STRETCHING:_____
_____
_____

DIET:_____
_____
_____

WEEKLY NOTES:
_____
_____
_____
_____
_____
_____

"Exercise in the morning before your brain figures out what you are doing."
- Anonymous

WEEK SIXTEEN: _____

MONDAY

CARDIO:_____
_____
_____

STRENGTH:_____
_____
_____

STRETCHING:_____
_____
_____

DIET:_____
_____
_____

TUESDAY

CARDIO:_____
_____
_____

STRENGTH:_____
_____
_____

STRETCHING:_____
_____
_____

DIET:_____
_____
_____

WEDNESDAY

CARDIO:_____
_____
_____

STRENGTH:_____
_____
_____

STRETCHING:_____

_____

_____

DIET:_____

_____

_____

_____

THURSDAY

CARDIO:_____

_____

_____

STRENGTH:_____

_____

_____

STRETCHING:_____

_____

_____

DIET:_____

_____

_____

FRIDAY

CARDIO:_____

_____

_____

STRENGTH:_____

_____

_____

STRETCHING:_____

_____

_____

DIET:_____

_____

_____

SATURDAY

CARDIO:_____
_____
_____

STRENGTH:_____
_____
_____

STRETCHING:_____
_____
_____

DIET:_____
_____
_____

SUNDAY

CARDIO:_____
_____
_____

STRENGTH:_____
_____
_____

STRETCHING:_____
_____
_____

DIET:_____
_____
_____

WEEKLY NOTES:
_____
_____
_____
_____
_____
_____
_____

"Family, nature, and health all go together." – Olivia Newton-John

WEEK SEVENTEEN: _____

MONDAY

CARDIO:_____
_____
_____

STRENGTH:_____
_____
_____

STRETCHING:_____
_____
_____

DIET:_____
_____
_____

TUESDAY

CARDIO:_____
_____
_____

STRENGTH:_____
_____
_____

STRETCHING:_____
_____
_____

DIET:_____
_____
_____

WEDNESDAY

CARDIO:_____
_____
_____

STRENGTH:_____
_____
_____

STRETCHING:_____
_____
_____

DIET:_____
_____
_____
_____

THURSDAY

CARDIO:_____
_____
_____

STRENGTH:_____
_____
_____

STRETCHING:_____
_____
_____

DIET:_____
_____
_____

FRIDAY

CARDIO:_____
_____
_____

STRENGTH:_____
_____
_____

STRETCHING:_____
_____
_____

DIET:_____
_____
_____

SATURDAY

CARDIO:_____
_____
_____

STRENGTH:_____
_____
_____

STRETCHING:_____
_____
_____

DIET:_____
_____
_____

SUNDAY

CARDIO:_____
_____
_____

STRENGTH:_____
_____
_____

STRETCHING:_____
_____
_____

DIET:_____
_____
_____

WEEKLY NOTES:
_____
_____
_____
_____
_____
_____

"At first they'll ask you why you're doing it and then they'll ask you how you did it." - Anonymous

WEEK EIGHTEEN: _____

MONDAY

CARDIO:_____
_____
_____

STRENGTH:_____
_____
_____

STRETCHING:_____
_____
_____

DIET:_____
_____
_____

TUESDAY

CARDIO:_____
_____
_____

STRENGTH:_____
_____
_____

STRETCHING:_____
_____
_____

DIET:_____
_____
_____

WEDNESDAY

CARDIO:_____
_____
_____

STRENGTH:_____
_____
_____

STRETCHING:_____

_____

_____

DIET:_____

_____

_____

_____

THURSDAY

CARDIO:_____

_____

_____

STRENGTH:_____

_____

_____

STRETCHING:_____

_____

_____

DIET:_____

_____

_____

FRIDAY

CARDIO:_____

_____

_____

STRENGTH:_____

_____

_____

STRETCHING:_____

_____

_____

DIET:_____

_____

_____

SATURDAY

CARDIO:_____
_____
_____

STRENGTH:_____
_____
_____

STRETCHING:_____
_____
_____

DIET:_____
_____
_____

SUNDAY

CARDIO:_____
_____
_____

STRENGTH:_____
_____
_____

STRETCHING:_____
_____
_____

DIET:_____
_____

WEEKLY NOTES:
_____
_____
_____
_____
_____
_____

"Make one healthy choice. Then make another one." – Sparkpeople.com

WEEK NINETEEN: _____

MONDAY

CARDIO:_____
_____
_____

STRENGTH:_____
_____
_____

STRETCHING:_____
_____
_____

DIET:_____
_____
_____

TUESDAY

CARDIO:_____
_____
_____

STRENGTH:_____
_____
_____

STRETCHING:_____
_____
_____

DIET:_____
_____
_____

WEDNESDAY

CARDIO:_____
_____
_____

STRENGTH:_____
_____
_____

STRETCHING:_____
_____
_____

DIET:_____
_____
_____
_____

THURSDAY

CARDIO:_____
_____
_____

STRENGTH:_____
_____
_____

STRETCHING:_____
_____
_____

DIET:_____
_____
_____

FRIDAY

CARDIO:_____
_____
_____

STRENGTH:_____
_____
_____

STRETCHING:_____
_____
_____

DIET:_____
_____
_____

SATURDAY

CARDIO:_____
_____
_____

STRENGTH:_____
_____
_____

STRETCHING:_____
_____
_____

DIET:_____
_____
_____

SUNDAY

CARDIO:_____
_____
_____

STRENGTH:_____
_____
_____

STRETCHING:_____
_____
_____

DIET:_____
_____
_____

WEEKLY NOTES:
_____
_____
_____
_____
_____
_____

"If you keep good food in your fridge, you will eat good food."
- Errick McAdams

WEEK TWENTY: _____

MONDAY

CARDIO:_____
_____
_____

STRENGTH:_____
_____
_____

STRETCHING:_____
_____
_____

DIET:_____
_____
_____

TUESDAY

CARDIO:_____
_____
_____

STRENGTH:_____
_____
_____

STRETCHING:_____
_____
_____

DIET:_____
_____
_____

WEDNESDAY

CARDIO:_____
_____
_____

STRENGTH:_____
_____
_____

STRETCHING:_____
_____
_____

DIET:_____
_____
_____
_____

THURSDAY

CARDIO:_____
_____
_____

STRENGTH:_____
_____
_____

STRETCHING:_____
_____
_____

DIET:_____
_____
_____

FRIDAY

CARDIO:_____
_____
_____

STRENGTH:_____
_____
_____

STRETCHING:_____
_____
_____

DIET:_____
_____
_____

SATURDAY

CARDIO:_____
_____
_____

STRENGTH:_____
_____
_____

STRETCHING:_____
_____
_____

DIET:_____
_____
_____

SUNDAY

CARDIO:_____
_____
_____

STRENGTH:_____
_____
_____

STRETCHING:_____
_____
_____

DIET:_____
_____
_____

WEEKLY NOTES:
_____
_____
_____
_____
_____
_____
_____

"It's all about making healthy habits, rather than restrictions." – a Weight Loss Blog

WEEK TWENTY ONE: _____

MONDAY

CARDIO:_____
_____
_____

STRENGTH:_____
_____
_____

STRETCHING:_____
_____
_____

DIET:_____
_____
_____

TUESDAY

CARDIO:_____
_____
_____

STRENGTH:_____
_____
_____

STRETCHING:_____
_____
_____

DIET:_____
_____
_____

WEDNESDAY

CARDIO:_____
_____
_____

STRENGTH:_____
_____
_____

STRETCHING:_____
_____
_____

DIET:_____
_____
_____
_____

THURSDAY

CARDIO:_____
_____
_____

STRENGTH:_____
_____
_____

STRETCHING:_____
_____
_____

DIET:_____
_____
_____

FRIDAY

CARDIO:_____
_____
_____

STRENGTH:_____
_____
_____

STRETCHING:_____
_____
_____

DIET:_____
_____
_____

SATURDAY

CARDIO:_____
_____
_____

STRENGTH:_____
_____
_____

STRETCHING:_____
_____
_____

DIET:_____
_____
_____

SUNDAY

CARDIO:_____
_____
_____

STRENGTH:_____
_____
_____

STRETCHING:_____
_____
_____

DIET:_____
_____
_____

WEEKLY NOTES:
_____
_____
_____
_____
_____
_____

"Nobody can do it for you, you have to do it yourself."
- Myweightlossdream.co.uk

WEEK TWENTY TWO: _____

MONDAY

CARDIO:_____
_____
_____

STRENGTH:_____
_____
_____

STRETCHING:_____
_____
_____

DIET:_____
_____
_____

TUESDAY

CARDIO:_____
_____
_____

STRENGTH:_____
_____
_____

STRETCHING:_____
_____
_____

DIET:_____
_____
_____

WEDNESDAY

CARDIO:_____
_____
_____

STRENGTH:_____
_____
_____

STRETCHING:_____
_____
_____

DIET:_____
_____
_____
_____

THURSDAY

CARDIO:_____
_____
_____

STRENGTH:_____
_____
_____

STRETCHING:_____
_____
_____

DIET:_____
_____
_____

FRIDAY

CARDIO:_____
_____
_____

STRENGTH:_____
_____
_____

STRETCHING:_____
_____
_____

DIET:_____
_____
_____

SATURDAY

CARDIO:_____
_____
_____

STRENGTH:_____
_____
_____

STRETCHING:_____
_____
_____

DIET:_____
_____
_____

SUNDAY

CARDIO:_____
_____
_____

STRENGTH:_____
_____
_____

STRETCHING:_____
_____
_____

DIET:_____
_____
_____

WEEKLY NOTES:
_____
_____
_____
_____
_____
_____

"The greatest medicine of all is to teach people how not to need it."
– Familyhealthchiropractic.com

WEEK TWENTY THREE: _____

MONDAY

CARDIO:_____
_____
_____

STRENGTH:_____
_____
_____

STRETCHING:_____
_____
_____

DIET:_____
_____
_____

TUESDAY

CARDIO:_____
_____
_____

STRENGTH:_____
_____
_____

STRETCHING:_____
_____
_____

DIET:_____
_____
_____

WEDNESDAY

CARDIO:_____
_____
_____

STRENGTH:_____
_____
_____

STRETCHING:_____

_____

_____

DIET:_____

_____

_____

_____

THURSDAY

CARDIO:_____

_____

_____

STRENGTH:_____

_____

_____

STRETCHING:_____

_____

_____

DIET:_____

_____

_____

FRIDAY

CARDIO:_____

_____

_____

STRENGTH:_____

_____

_____

STRETCHING:_____

_____

_____

DIET:_____

_____

_____

SATURDAY

CARDIO:_____
_____
_____

STRENGTH:_____
_____
_____

STRETCHING:_____
_____
_____

DIET:_____
_____
_____

SUNDAY

CARDIO:_____
_____
_____

STRENGTH:_____
_____
_____

STRETCHING:_____
_____
_____

DIET:_____
_____
_____

WEEKLY NOTES:
_____
_____
_____
_____
_____
_____
_____

"Early to bed, early to rise makes a man healthy, wealthy, and wise."
- Benjamin Franklin

WEEK TWENTY FOUR: _____

MONDAY

CARDIO:_____
_____
_____

STRENGTH:_____
_____
_____

STRETCHING:_____
_____
_____

DIET:_____
_____
_____

TUESDAY

CARDIO:_____
_____
_____

STRENGTH:_____
_____
_____

STRETCHING:_____
_____
_____

DIET:_____
_____
_____

WEDNESDAY

CARDIO:_____
_____
_____

STRENGTH:_____
_____
_____

STRETCHING:_____
_____
_____

DIET:_____
_____
_____

THURSDAY

CARDIO:_____
_____
_____

STRENGTH:_____
_____
_____

STRETCHING:_____
_____
_____

DIET:_____
_____
_____

FRIDAY

CARDIO:_____
_____
_____

STRENGTH:_____
_____
_____

STRETCHING:_____
_____
_____

DIET:_____
_____
_____

SATURDAY

CARDIO:_____
_____
_____

STRENGTH:_____
_____
_____

STRETCHING:_____
_____
_____

DIET:_____
_____
_____

SUNDAY

CARDIO:_____
_____
_____

STRENGTH:_____
_____
_____

STRETCHING:_____
_____
_____

DIET:_____
_____
_____

WEEKLY NOTES:
_____
_____
_____
_____
_____
_____

"Healthy isn't a goal. It's a way of living." - Young Wild + Fit Blogspot

WEEK TWENTY FIVE: _____

MONDAY

CARDIO:_____
_____
_____

STRENGTH:_____
_____
_____

STRETCHING:_____
_____
_____

DIET:_____
_____
_____

TUESDAY

CARDIO:_____
_____
_____

STRENGTH:_____
_____
_____

STRETCHING:_____
_____
_____

DIET:_____
_____
_____

WEDNESDAY

CARDIO:_____
_____
_____

STRENGTH:_____
_____
_____

STRETCHING:_____
_____
_____

DIET:_____
_____
_____
_____

THURSDAY

CARDIO:_____
_____
_____

STRENGTH:_____
_____
_____

STRETCHING:_____
_____
_____

DIET:_____
_____
_____

FRIDAY

CARDIO:_____
_____
_____

STRENGTH:_____
_____
_____

STRETCHING:_____
_____
_____

DIET:_____
_____
_____

SATURDAY

CARDIO:_____
_____
_____

STRENGTH:_____
_____
_____

STRETCHING:_____
_____
_____

DIET:_____
_____
_____

SUNDAY

CARDIO:_____
_____
_____

STRENGTH:_____
_____
_____

STRETCHING:_____
_____
_____

DIET:_____
_____
_____

WEEKLY NOTES:
_____
_____
_____
_____
_____
_____

"When you feel like quitting, ask yourself why you started."
- Young Wild + Fit Blogspot

WEEK TWENTY SIX: _____

MONDAY

CARDIO:_____
_____
_____

STRENGTH:_____
_____
_____

STRETCHING:_____
_____
_____

DIET:_____
_____
_____

TUESDAY

CARDIO:_____
_____
_____

STRENGTH:_____
_____
_____

STRETCHING:_____
_____
_____

DIET:_____
_____
_____

WEDNESDAY

CARDIO:_____
_____
_____

STRENGTH:_____
_____
_____

STRETCHING:_____

_____

_____

DIET:_____

_____

_____

_____

THURSDAY

CARDIO:_____

_____

_____

STRENGTH:_____

_____

_____

STRETCHING:_____

_____

_____

DIET:_____

_____

_____

FRIDAY

CARDIO:_____

_____

_____

STRENGTH:_____

_____

_____

STRETCHING:_____

_____

_____

DIET:_____

_____

_____

SATURDAY

CARDIO:_____
_____
_____

STRENGTH:_____
_____
_____

STRETCHING:_____
_____
_____

DIET:_____
_____
_____

SUNDAY

CARDIO:_____
_____
_____

STRENGTH:_____
_____
_____

STRETCHING:_____
_____
_____

DIET:_____
_____
_____

WEEKLY NOTES:
_____
_____
_____
_____
_____
_____

"I'm not telling you it's going to be easy – I'm telling you it's going to be worth it." – Art Williams

WEEK TWENTY SEVEN: _____

MONDAY

CARDIO:_____
_____
_____

STRENGTH:_____
_____
_____

STRETCHING:_____
_____
_____

DIET:_____
_____
_____

TUESDAY

CARDIO:_____
_____
_____

STRENGTH:_____
_____
_____

STRETCHING:_____
_____
_____

DIET:_____
_____
_____

WEDNESDAY

CARDIO:_____
_____
_____

STRENGTH:_____
_____
_____

STRETCHING:_____
_____
_____

DIET:_____
_____
_____
_____

THURSDAY

CARDIO:_____
_____
_____

STRENGTH:_____
_____
_____

STRETCHING:_____
_____
_____

DIET:_____
_____
_____

FRIDAY

CARDIO:_____
_____
_____

STRENGTH:_____
_____
_____

STRETCHING:_____
_____
_____

DIET:_____
_____
_____

SATURDAY

CARDIO:_____
_____
_____

STRENGTH:_____
_____
_____

STRETCHING:_____
_____
_____

DIET:_____
_____
_____

SUNDAY

CARDIO:_____
_____
_____

STRENGTH:_____
_____
_____

STRETCHING:_____
_____
_____

DIET:_____
_____
_____

WEEKLY NOTES:
_____
_____
_____
_____
_____
_____

"Life does not get better by chance it gets better by change." – Jim Rohn

WEEK TWENTY EIGHT: _____

MONDAY

CARDIO:_____
_____
_____

STRENGTH:_____
_____
_____

STRETCHING:_____
_____
_____

DIET:_____
_____
_____

TUESDAY

CARDIO:_____
_____
_____

STRENGTH:_____
_____
_____

STRETCHING:_____
_____
_____

DIET:_____
_____
_____

WEDNESDAY

CARDIO:_____
_____
_____

STRENGTH:_____
_____
_____

STRETCHING:_____

_____

_____

DIET:_____

_____

_____

_____

THURSDAY

CARDIO:_____

_____

_____

STRENGTH:_____

_____

_____

STRETCHING:_____

_____

_____

DIET:_____

_____

_____

FRIDAY

CARDIO:_____

_____

_____

STRENGTH:_____

_____

_____

STRETCHING:_____

_____

_____

DIET:_____

_____

_____

SATURDAY

CARDIO:_____

_____

_____

STRENGTH:_____

_____

_____

STRETCHING:_____

_____

_____

DIET:_____

_____

_____

SUNDAY

CARDIO:_____

_____

_____

STRENGTH:_____

_____

_____

STRETCHING:_____

_____

_____

DIET:_____

_____

WEEKLY NOTES:

_____

_____

_____

_____

_____

_____

_____

"Those who think they have no time for healthy eating will sooner or later have to make time for illness." – B-Wellness Fitness & Style

WEEK TWENTY NINE: _____

MONDAY

CARDIO:_____
_____
_____

STRENGTH:_____
_____
_____

STRETCHING:_____
_____
_____

DIET:_____
_____
_____

TUESDAY

CARDIO:_____
_____
_____

STRENGTH:_____
_____
_____

STRETCHING:_____
_____
_____

DIET:_____
_____
_____

WEDNESDAY

CARDIO:_____
_____
_____

STRENGTH:_____
_____
_____

STRETCHING:_____

_____

_____

DIET:_____

_____

_____

_____

THURSDAY

CARDIO:_____

_____

_____

STRENGTH:_____

_____

_____

STRETCHING:_____

_____

_____

DIET:_____

_____

_____

FRIDAY

CARDIO:_____

_____

_____

STRENGTH:_____

_____

_____

STRETCHING:_____

_____

_____

DIET:_____

_____

_____

SATURDAY

CARDIO:_____
_____
_____

STRENGTH:_____
_____
_____

STRETCHING:_____
_____
_____

DIET:_____
_____
_____

SUNDAY

CARDIO:_____
_____
_____

STRENGTH:_____
_____
_____

STRETCHING:_____
_____
_____

DIET:_____
_____
_____

WEEKLY NOTES:
_____
_____
_____
_____
_____
_____

"The part can never be well unless the whole is well." - Plato

WEEK THIRTY: _____

MONDAY

CARDIO:_____
_____
_____

STRENGTH:_____
_____
_____

STRETCHING:_____
_____
_____

DIET:_____
_____
_____

TUESDAY

CARDIO:_____
_____
_____

STRENGTH:_____
_____
_____

STRETCHING:_____
_____
_____

DIET:_____
_____
_____

WEDNESDAY

CARDIO:_____
_____
_____

STRENGTH:_____
_____
_____

STRETCHING:_____

_____

_____

DIET:_____

_____

_____

_____

THURSDAY

CARDIO:_____

_____

_____

STRENGTH:_____

_____

_____

STRETCHING:_____

_____

_____

DIET:_____

_____

_____

FRIDAY

CARDIO:_____

_____

_____

STRENGTH:_____

_____

_____

STRETCHING:_____

_____

_____

DIET:_____

_____

_____

SATURDAY

CARDIO:_____
_____
_____

STRENGTH:_____
_____
_____

STRETCHING:_____
_____
_____

DIET:_____
_____
_____

SUNDAY

CARDIO:_____
_____
_____

STRENGTH:_____
_____
_____

STRETCHING:_____
_____
_____

DIET:_____
_____
_____

WEEKLY NOTES:
_____
_____
_____
_____
_____
_____

"Healing is a matter of time but sometimes it is also a matter of opportunity."
- Hippocrates

WEEK THIRTY ONE: _____

MONDAY

CARDIO:_____
_____
_____

STRENGTH:_____
_____
_____

STRETCHING:_____
_____
_____

DIET:_____
_____
_____

TUESDAY

CARDIO:_____
_____
_____

STRENGTH:_____
_____
_____

STRETCHING:_____
_____
_____

DIET:_____
_____
_____

WEDNESDAY

CARDIO:_____
_____
_____

STRENGTH:_____
_____
_____

STRETCHING:_____
_____
_____

DIET:_____
_____
_____
_____

THURSDAY

CARDIO:_____
_____
_____

STRENGTH:_____
_____
_____

STRETCHING:_____
_____
_____

DIET:_____
_____
_____

FRIDAY

CARDIO:_____
_____
_____

STRENGTH:_____
_____
_____

STRETCHING:_____
_____
_____

DIET:_____
_____
_____

SATURDAY

CARDIO:_____
_____
_____

STRENGTH:_____
_____
_____

STRETCHING:_____
_____
_____

DIET:_____
_____
_____

SUNDAY

CARDIO:_____
_____
_____

STRENGTH:_____
_____
_____

STRETCHING:_____
_____
_____

DIET:_____
_____
_____

WEEKLY NOTES:
_____
_____
_____
_____
_____
_____

"Sleep is that golden chain that ties health and our bodies together."
- Thomas Dekker

WEEK THIRTY TWO: _____

MONDAY

CARDIO:_____
_____
_____

STRENGTH:_____
_____
_____

STRETCHING:_____
_____
_____

DIET:_____
_____
_____

TUESDAY

CARDIO:_____
_____
_____

STRENGTH:_____
_____
_____

STRETCHING:_____
_____
_____

DIET:_____
_____
_____

WEDNESDAY

CARDIO:_____
_____
_____

STRENGTH:_____
_____
_____

STRETCHING:_____

_____

_____

DIET:_____

_____

_____

_____

THURSDAY

CARDIO:_____

_____

_____

STRENGTH:_____

_____

_____

STRETCHING:_____

_____

_____

DIET:_____

_____

_____

FRIDAY

CARDIO:_____

_____

_____

STRENGTH:_____

_____

_____

STRETCHING:_____

_____

_____

DIET:_____

_____

_____

SATURDAY

CARDIO:_____
_____
_____

STRENGTH:_____
_____
_____

STRETCHING:_____
_____
_____

DIET:_____
_____
_____

SUNDAY

CARDIO:_____
_____
_____

STRENGTH:_____
_____
_____

STRETCHING:_____
_____
_____

DIET:_____
_____
_____

WEEKLY NOTES:
_____
_____
_____
_____
_____
_____

"Health is not valued until sickness comes." – Thomas Fuller

WEEK THIRTY THREE: _____

MONDAY

CARDIO:_____
_____
_____

STRENGTH:_____
_____
_____

STRETCHING:_____
_____
_____

DIET:_____
_____
_____

TUESDAY

CARDIO:_____
_____
_____

STRENGTH:_____
_____
_____

STRETCHING:_____
_____
_____

DIET:_____
_____
_____

WEDNESDAY

CARDIO:_____
_____
_____

STRENGTH:_____
_____
_____

STRETCHING:_____

_____

_____

DIET:_____

_____

_____

_____

THURSDAY

CARDIO:_____

_____

_____

STRENGTH:_____

_____

_____

STRETCHING:_____

_____

_____

DIET:_____

_____

_____

FRIDAY

CARDIO:_____

_____

_____

STRENGTH:_____

_____

_____

STRETCHING:_____

_____

_____

DIET:_____

_____

_____

SATURDAY

CARDIO:_____
_____
_____

STRENGTH:_____
_____
_____

STRETCHING:_____
_____
_____

DIET:_____
_____
_____

SUNDAY

CARDIO:_____
_____
_____

STRENGTH:_____
_____
_____

STRETCHING:_____
_____
_____

DIET:_____
_____
_____

WEEKLY NOTES:
_____
_____
_____
_____
_____
_____

"Water, air, and cleanness are the chief articles in my pharmacy."
- Napolean Bonaparte

WEEK THIRTY FOUR: _____

MONDAY

CARDIO:_____
_____
_____

STRENGTH:_____
_____
_____

STRETCHING:_____
_____
_____

DIET:_____
_____
_____

TUESDAY

CARDIO:_____
_____
_____

STRENGTH:_____
_____
_____

STRETCHING:_____
_____
_____

DIET:_____
_____
_____

WEDNESDAY

CARDIO:_____
_____
_____

STRENGTH:_____
_____
_____

STRETCHING:_____

_____

_____

DIET:_____

_____

_____

_____

THURSDAY

CARDIO:_____

_____

_____

STRENGTH:_____

_____

_____

STRETCHING:_____

_____

_____

DIET:_____

_____

_____

FRIDAY

CARDIO:_____

_____

_____

STRENGTH:_____

_____

_____

STRETCHING:_____

_____

_____

DIET:_____

_____

_____

SATURDAY

CARDIO:_____

_____

_____

STRENGTH:_____

_____

_____

STRETCHING:_____

_____

_____

DIET:_____

_____

_____

SUNDAY

CARDIO:_____

_____

_____

STRENGTH:_____

_____

_____

STRETCHING:_____

_____

_____

DIET:_____

_____

_____

WEEKLY NOTES:

_____

_____

_____

_____

_____

_____

"Cheerfulness is the best promoter of health and is as friendly to the mind as to the body." – Joseph Addison

WEEK THIRTY FIVE: _____

MONDAY

CARDIO:_____
_____
_____

STRENGTH:_____
_____
_____

STRETCHING:_____
_____
_____

DIET:_____
_____
_____

TUESDAY

CARDIO:_____
_____
_____

STRENGTH:_____
_____
_____

STRETCHING:_____
_____
_____

DIET:_____
_____
_____

WEDNESDAY

CARDIO:_____
_____
_____

STRENGTH:_____
_____
_____

STRETCHING:_____

_____

_____

DIET:_____

_____

_____

_____

THURSDAY

CARDIO:_____

_____

_____

STRENGTH:_____

_____

_____

STRETCHING:_____

_____

_____

DIET:_____

_____

_____

FRIDAY

CARDIO:_____

_____

_____

STRENGTH:_____

_____

_____

STRETCHING:_____

_____

_____

DIET:_____

_____

_____

SATURDAY

CARDIO:_____
_____
_____

STRENGTH:_____
_____
_____

STRETCHING:_____
_____
_____

DIET:_____
_____
_____

SUNDAY

CARDIO:_____
_____
_____

STRENGTH:_____
_____
_____

STRETCHING:_____
_____
_____

DIET:_____
_____
_____

WEEKLY NOTES:
_____
_____
_____
_____
_____
_____

"Happiness lies first of all in health." – George William Curtis

WEEK THIRTY SIX: _____

MONDAY

CARDIO:_____
_____
_____

STRENGTH:_____
_____
_____

STRETCHING:_____
_____
_____

DIET:_____
_____
_____

TUESDAY

CARDIO:_____
_____
_____

STRENGTH:_____
_____
_____

STRETCHING:_____
_____
_____

DIET:_____
_____
_____

WEDNESDAY

CARDIO:_____
_____
_____

STRENGTH:_____
_____
_____

STRETCHING:_____
_____
_____

DIET:_____
_____
_____
_____

THURSDAY

CARDIO:_____
_____
_____

STRENGTH:_____
_____
_____

STRETCHING:_____
_____
_____

DIET:_____
_____
_____

FRIDAY

CARDIO:_____
_____
_____

STRENGTH:_____
_____
_____

STRETCHING:_____
_____
_____

DIET:_____
_____
_____

SATURDAY

CARDIO:_____
_____
_____

STRENGTH:_____
_____
_____

STRETCHING:_____
_____
_____

DIET:_____
_____
_____

SUNDAY

CARDIO:_____
_____
_____

STRENGTH:_____
_____
_____

STRETCHING:_____
_____
_____

DIET:_____
_____
_____

WEEKLY NOTES:
_____
_____
_____
_____
_____
_____

"It takes more than just a good looking body. You've got to have the heart and soul to go with it." - Epictetus

WEEK THIRTY SEVEN: _____

MONDAY

CARDIO:_____
_____
_____

STRENGTH:_____
_____
_____

STRETCHING:_____
_____
_____

DIET:_____
_____
_____

TUESDAY

CARDIO:_____
_____
_____

STRENGTH:_____
_____
_____

STRETCHING:_____
_____
_____

DIET:_____
_____
_____

WEDNESDAY

CARDIO:_____
_____
_____

STRENGTH:_____
_____
_____

STRETCHING:_____
_____
_____

DIET:_____
_____
_____
_____

THURSDAY

CARDIO:_____
_____
_____

STRENGTH:_____
_____
_____

STRETCHING:_____
_____
_____

DIET:_____
_____
_____

FRIDAY

CARDIO:_____
_____
_____

STRENGTH:_____
_____
_____

STRETCHING:_____
_____
_____

DIET:_____
_____
_____

SATURDAY

CARDIO:_____
_____
_____

STRENGTH:_____
_____
_____

STRETCHING:_____
_____
_____

DIET:_____
_____
_____

SUNDAY

CARDIO:_____
_____
_____

STRENGTH:_____
_____
_____

STRETCHING:_____
_____
_____

DIET:_____
_____
_____

WEEKLY NOTES:
_____
_____
_____
_____
_____
_____

"I do not think about being beautiful. What I devote most of my time to is being healthy." – Ann Bancroft

WEEK THIRTY EIGHT: _____

MONDAY

CARDIO:_____
_____
_____

STRENGTH:_____
_____
_____

STRETCHING:_____
_____
_____

DIET:_____
_____
_____

TUESDAY

CARDIO:_____
_____
_____

STRENGTH:_____
_____
_____

STRETCHING:_____
_____
_____

DIET:_____
_____
_____

WEDNESDAY

CARDIO:_____
_____
_____

STRENGTH:_____
_____
_____

STRETCHING:_____

_____

_____

DIET:_____

_____

_____

_____

THURSDAY

CARDIO:_____

_____

_____

STRENGTH:_____

_____

_____

STRETCHING:_____

_____

_____

DIET:_____

_____

_____

FRIDAY

CARDIO:_____

_____

_____

STRENGTH:_____

_____

_____

STRETCHING:_____

_____

_____

DIET:_____

_____

_____

SATURDAY

CARDIO:_____
_____
_____

STRENGTH:_____
_____
_____

STRETCHING:_____
_____
_____

DIET:_____
_____
_____

SUNDAY

CARDIO:_____
_____
_____

STRENGTH:_____
_____
_____

STRETCHING:_____
_____
_____

DIET:_____
_____
_____

WEEKLY NOTES:
_____
_____
_____
_____
_____
_____

"Good health and good sense are two of life's greatest blessings." – Publilius Syrus

WEEK THIRTY NINE: _____

MONDAY

CARDIO:_____
_____
_____

STRENGTH:_____
_____
_____

STRETCHING:_____
_____
_____

DIET:_____
_____
_____

TUESDAY

CARDIO:_____
_____
_____

STRENGTH:_____
_____
_____

STRETCHING:_____
_____
_____

DIET:_____
_____
_____

WEDNESDAY

CARDIO:_____
_____
_____

STRENGTH:_____
_____
_____

STRETCHING:_____
_____
_____

DIET:_____
_____
_____
_____

THURSDAY

CARDIO:_____
_____
_____

STRENGTH:_____
_____
_____

STRETCHING:_____
_____
_____

DIET:_____
_____
_____

FRIDAY

CARDIO:_____
_____
_____

STRENGTH:_____
_____
_____

STRETCHING:_____
_____
_____

DIET:_____
_____
_____

SATURDAY

CARDIO:_____
_____
_____

STRENGTH:_____
_____
_____

STRETCHING:_____
_____
_____

DIET:_____
_____
_____

SUNDAY

CARDIO:_____
_____
_____

STRENGTH:_____
_____
_____

STRETCHING:_____
_____
_____

DIET:_____
_____
_____

WEEKLY NOTES:
_____
_____
_____
_____
_____
_____

"To enjoy the glow of good health, you must exercise." – Gene Tunney

WEEK FORTY: _____

MONDAY

CARDIO:_____
_____
_____

STRENGTH:_____
_____
_____

STRETCHING:_____
_____
_____

DIET:_____
_____
_____

TUESDAY

CARDIO:_____
_____
_____

STRENGTH:_____
_____
_____

STRETCHING:_____
_____
_____

DIET:_____
_____
_____

WEDNESDAY

CARDIO:_____
_____
_____

STRENGTH:_____
_____
_____

STRETCHING:_____
_____
_____

DIET:_____
_____
_____
_____

THURSDAY

CARDIO:_____
_____
_____

STRENGTH:_____
_____
_____

STRETCHING:_____
_____
_____

DIET:_____
_____
_____

FRIDAY

CARDIO:_____
_____
_____

STRENGTH:_____
_____
_____

STRETCHING:_____
_____
_____

DIET:_____
_____
_____

SATURDAY

CARDIO:_____
_____
_____

STRENGTH:_____
_____
_____

STRETCHING:_____
_____
_____

DIET:_____
_____
_____

SUNDAY

CARDIO:_____
_____
_____

STRENGTH:_____
_____
_____

STRETCHING:_____
_____
_____

DIET:_____
_____

WEEKLY NOTES:
_____
_____
_____
_____
_____
_____

"It is better to lose health like a spendthrift than to waste it like a miser."
- Robert Louis Stevenson

WEEK FORTY ONE: _____

MONDAY

CARDIO:_____
_____
_____

STRENGTH:_____
_____
_____

STRETCHING:_____
_____
_____

DIET:_____
_____
_____

TUESDAY

CARDIO:_____
_____
_____

STRENGTH:_____
_____
_____

STRETCHING:_____
_____
_____

DIET:_____
_____
_____

WEDNESDAY

CARDIO:_____
_____
_____

STRENGTH:_____
_____
_____

STRETCHING:_____
_____
_____

DIET:_____
_____
_____
_____

THURSDAY

CARDIO:_____
_____
_____

STRENGTH:_____
_____
_____

STRETCHING:_____
_____
_____

DIET:_____
_____
_____

FRIDAY

CARDIO:_____
_____
_____

STRENGTH:_____
_____
_____

STRETCHING:_____
_____
_____

DIET:_____
_____
_____

SATURDAY

CARDIO:_____
_____
_____

STRENGTH:_____
_____
_____

STRETCHING:_____
_____
_____

DIET:_____
_____
_____

SUNDAY

CARDIO:_____
_____
_____

STRENGTH:_____
_____
_____

STRETCHING:_____
_____
_____

DIET:_____
_____

WEEKLY NOTES:
_____
_____
_____
_____
_____
_____

"In health there is freedom. Health is the first of all liberties."
– Henri Frederic Amiel

WEEK FORTY TWO: _____

MONDAY

CARDIO:_____
_____
_____

STRENGTH:_____
_____
_____

STRETCHING:_____
_____
_____

DIET:_____
_____
_____

TUESDAY

CARDIO:_____
_____
_____

STRENGTH:_____
_____
_____

STRETCHING:_____
_____
_____

DIET:_____
_____
_____

WEDNESDAY

CARDIO:_____
_____
_____

STRENGTH:_____
_____
_____

STRETCHING:_____
_____
_____

DIET:_____
_____
_____
_____

THURSDAY

CARDIO:_____
_____
_____

STRENGTH:_____
_____
_____

STRETCHING:_____
_____
_____

DIET:_____
_____
_____

FRIDAY

CARDIO:_____
_____
_____

STRENGTH:_____
_____
_____

STRETCHING:_____
_____
_____

DIET:_____
_____
_____

SATURDAY

CARDIO:_____

_____

_____

STRENGTH:_____

_____

_____

STRETCHING:_____

_____

_____

DIET:_____

_____

_____

SUNDAY

CARDIO:_____

_____

_____

STRENGTH:_____

_____

_____

STRETCHING:_____

_____

_____

DIET:_____

_____

_____

WEEKLY NOTES:

_____

_____

_____

_____

_____

_____

"I have no regrets. I have my health." – Naomi Campbell

WEEK FORTY THREE: _____

MONDAY

CARDIO:_____
_____
_____

STRENGTH:_____
_____
_____

STRETCHING:_____
_____
_____

DIET:_____
_____
_____

TUESDAY

CARDIO:_____
_____
_____

STRENGTH:_____
_____
_____

STRETCHING:_____
_____
_____

DIET:_____
_____
_____

WEDNESDAY

CARDIO:_____
_____
_____

STRENGTH:_____
_____
_____

STRETCHING:_____
_____
_____

DIET:_____
_____
_____
_____

THURSDAY

CARDIO:_____
_____
_____

STRENGTH:_____
_____
_____

STRETCHING:_____
_____
_____

DIET:_____
_____
_____

FRIDAY

CARDIO:_____
_____
_____

STRENGTH:_____
_____
_____

STRETCHING:_____
_____
_____

DIET:_____
_____
_____

SATURDAY

CARDIO:_____
_____
_____

STRENGTH:_____
_____
_____

STRETCHING:_____
_____
_____

DIET:_____
_____
_____

SUNDAY

CARDIO:_____
_____
_____

STRENGTH:_____
_____
_____

STRETCHING:_____
_____
_____

DIET:_____
_____
_____

WEEKLY NOTES:
_____
_____
_____
_____
_____
_____
_____

"Leave all the afternoon for exercise and recreation, which are as necessary as reading. I will rather say more necessary because health is worth more than learning." – Thomas Jefferson

WEEK FORTY FOUR: _____

MONDAY

CARDIO:_____
_____
_____

STRENGTH:_____
_____
_____

STRETCHING:_____
_____
_____

DIET:_____
_____
_____

TUESDAY

CARDIO:_____
_____
_____

STRENGTH:_____
_____
_____

STRETCHING:_____
_____
_____

DIET:_____
_____
_____

WEDNESDAY

CARDIO:_____
_____
_____

STRENGTH:_____
_____
_____

STRETCHING:_____
_____
_____

DIET:_____
_____
_____
_____

THURSDAY

CARDIO:_____
_____
_____

STRENGTH:_____
_____
_____

STRETCHING:_____
_____
_____

DIET:_____
_____
_____

FRIDAY

CARDIO:_____
_____
_____

STRENGTH:_____
_____
_____

STRETCHING:_____
_____
_____

DIET:_____
_____
_____

SATURDAY

CARDIO:_____
_____
_____

STRENGTH:_____
_____
_____

STRETCHING:_____
_____
_____

DIET:_____
_____
_____

SUNDAY

CARDIO:_____
_____
_____

STRENGTH:_____
_____
_____

STRETCHING:_____
_____
_____

DIET:_____
_____
_____

WEEKLY NOTES:
_____
_____
_____
_____
_____
_____

"The body needs its rest, sleep is extremely important in any health regime. There should be 3 main things: eating, exercise and sleep. All 3 together in the right balance make for a truly healthy lifestyle." – Rohit Shetty

WEEK FORTY FIVE: _____

MONDAY

CARDIO:_____
_____
_____

STRENGTH:_____
_____
_____

STRETCHING:_____
_____
_____

DIET:_____
_____
_____

TUESDAY

CARDIO:_____
_____
_____

STRENGTH:_____
_____
_____

STRETCHING:_____
_____
_____

DIET:_____
_____
_____

WEDNESDAY

CARDIO:_____
_____
_____

STRENGTH:_____
_____
_____

STRETCHING:_____
_____
_____

DIET:_____
_____
_____
_____

THURSDAY

CARDIO:_____
_____
_____

STRENGTH:_____
_____
_____

STRETCHING:_____
_____
_____

DIET:_____
_____
_____

FRIDAY

CARDIO:_____
_____
_____

STRENGTH:_____
_____
_____

STRETCHING:_____
_____
_____

DIET:_____
_____
_____

SATURDAY

CARDIO:_____
_____
_____

STRENGTH:_____
_____
_____

STRETCHING:_____
_____
_____

DIET:_____
_____
_____

SUNDAY

CARDIO:_____
_____
_____

STRENGTH:_____
_____
_____

STRETCHING:_____
_____
_____

DIET:_____
_____
_____

WEEKLY NOTES:
_____
_____
_____
_____
_____
_____

"Cutting back on calories is not the answer to successful weight loss and successful health. You have to increase the quality of what you eat, not just reduce the quantity." – Joel Fuhrman

WEEK FORTY SIX: _____

MONDAY

CARDIO:_____
_____
_____

STRENGTH:_____
_____
_____

STRETCHING:_____
_____
_____

DIET:_____
_____
_____

TUESDAY

CARDIO:_____
_____
_____

STRENGTH:_____
_____
_____

STRETCHING:_____
_____
_____

DIET:_____
_____
_____

WEDNESDAY

CARDIO:_____
_____
_____

STRENGTH:_____
_____
_____

STRETCHING:_____
_____
_____

DIET:_____
_____
_____
_____

THURSDAY

CARDIO:_____
_____
_____

STRENGTH:_____
_____
_____

STRETCHING:_____
_____
_____

DIET:_____
_____
_____

FRIDAY

CARDIO:_____
_____
_____

STRENGTH:_____
_____
_____

STRETCHING:_____
_____
_____

DIET:_____
_____

SATURDAY

CARDIO:_____
_____
_____

STRENGTH:_____
_____
_____

STRETCHING:_____
_____
_____

DIET:_____
_____
_____

SUNDAY

CARDIO:_____
_____
_____

STRENGTH:_____
_____
_____

STRETCHING:_____
_____
_____

DIET:_____
_____
_____

WEEKLY NOTES:
_____
_____
_____
_____
_____
_____

"Exercise to stimulate, not to annihilate. The world wasn't formed in a day, and neither were we. Set small goals and build upon them." – Lee Haney

MONDAY

CARDIO:_____
_____
_____

STRENGTH:_____
_____
_____

STRETCHING:_____
_____
_____

DIET:_____
_____
_____

TUESDAY

CARDIO:_____
_____
_____

STRENGTH:_____
_____
_____

STRETCHING:_____
_____
_____

DIET:_____
_____
_____

WEDNESDAY

CARDIO:_____
_____
_____

STRENGTH:_____
_____
_____

STRETCHING:_____
_____
_____

DIET:_____
_____
_____
_____

THURSDAY

CARDIO:_____
_____
_____

STRENGTH:_____
_____
_____

STRETCHING:_____
_____
_____

DIET:_____
_____
_____

FRIDAY

CARDIO:_____
_____
_____

STRENGTH:_____
_____
_____

STRETCHING:_____
_____
_____

DIET:_____
_____
_____

SATURDAY

CARDIO:_____

_____

_____

STRENGTH:_____

_____

_____

STRETCHING:_____

_____

_____

DIET:_____

_____

_____

SUNDAY

CARDIO:_____

_____

_____

STRENGTH:_____

_____

_____

STRETCHING:_____

_____

_____

DIET:_____

_____

_____

WEEKLY NOTES:

_____

_____

_____

_____

_____

_____

"I like to embrace natural health. I try to get at least 8 hours of sleep, drinking a lot of water and exercising." – Tia Mowry

WEEK FORTY EIGHT: _____

MONDAY

CARDIO:_____
_____
_____

STRENGTH:_____
_____
_____

STRETCHING:_____
_____
_____

DIET:_____
_____
_____

TUESDAY

CARDIO:_____
_____
_____

STRENGTH:_____
_____
_____

STRETCHING:_____
_____
_____

DIET:_____
_____
_____

WEDNESDAY

CARDIO:_____
_____
_____

STRENGTH:_____
_____
_____

STRETCHING:_____

_____

_____

DIET:_____

_____

_____

_____

THURSDAY

CARDIO:_____

_____

_____

STRENGTH:_____

_____

_____

STRETCHING:_____

_____

_____

DIET:_____

_____

_____

FRIDAY

CARDIO:_____

_____

_____

STRENGTH:_____

_____

_____

STRETCHING:_____

_____

_____

DIET:_____

_____

_____

SATURDAY

CARDIO:_____
_____
_____

STRENGTH:_____
_____
_____

STRETCHING:_____
_____
_____

DIET:_____
_____
_____

SUNDAY

CARDIO:_____
_____
_____

STRENGTH:_____
_____
_____

STRETCHING:_____
_____
_____

DIET:_____
_____
_____

WEEKLY NOTES:
_____
_____
_____
_____
_____
_____

"The reason I exercise is for the quality of life I enjoy." – Kenneth H Cooper

WEEK FORTY NINE: _____

MONDAY

CARDIO:_____
_____
_____

STRENGTH:_____
_____
_____

STRETCHING:_____
_____
_____

DIET:_____
_____
_____

TUESDAY

CARDIO:_____
_____
_____

STRENGTH:_____
_____
_____

STRETCHING:_____
_____
_____

DIET:_____
_____

WEDNESDAY

CARDIO:_____
_____
_____

STRENGTH:_____
_____
_____

STRETCHING:_____
_____
_____

DIET:_____
_____
_____
_____

THURSDAY

CARDIO:_____
_____
_____

STRENGTH:_____
_____
_____

STRETCHING:_____
_____
_____

DIET:_____
_____
_____

FRIDAY

CARDIO:_____
_____
_____

STRENGTH:_____
_____
_____

STRETCHING:_____
_____
_____

DIET:_____
_____
_____

SATURDAY

CARDIO:_____
_____
_____

STRENGTH:_____
_____
_____

STRETCHING:_____
_____
_____

DIET:_____
_____
_____

SUNDAY

CARDIO:_____
_____
_____

STRENGTH:_____
_____
_____

STRETCHING:_____
_____
_____

DIET:_____
_____
_____

WEEKLY NOTES:
_____
_____
_____
_____
_____
_____

"A muscle is like a car. If you want it to run well early in the morning, you have to warm it up." – Florence Griffith Joyner

WEEK FIFTY: _____

MONDAY

CARDIO:_____
_____
_____

STRENGTH:_____
_____
_____

STRETCHING:_____
_____
_____

DIET:_____
_____
_____

TUESDAY

CARDIO:_____
_____
_____

STRENGTH:_____
_____
_____

STRETCHING:_____
_____
_____

DIET:_____
_____
_____

WEDNESDAY

CARDIO:_____
_____
_____

STRENGTH:_____
_____
_____

STRETCHING:_____
_____
_____

DIET:_____
_____
_____
_____

THURSDAY

CARDIO:_____
_____
_____

STRENGTH:_____
_____
_____

STRETCHING:_____
_____
_____

DIET:_____
_____
_____

FRIDAY

CARDIO:_____
_____
_____

STRENGTH:_____
_____
_____

STRETCHING:_____
_____
_____

DIET:_____
_____
_____

SATURDAY

CARDIO:_____

_____

_____

STRENGTH:_____

_____

_____

STRETCHING:_____

_____

_____

DIET:_____

_____

_____

SUNDAY

CARDIO:_____

_____

_____

STRENGTH:_____

_____

_____

STRETCHING:_____

_____

_____

DIET:_____

_____

WEEKLY NOTES:

_____

_____

_____

_____

_____

_____

"Exercise is amazing, from the inside out. I feel so alive and have more energy." – Vanessa Hudgens

WEEK FIFTY ONE: _____

MONDAY

CARDIO:_____
_____
_____

STRENGTH:_____
_____
_____

STRETCHING:_____
_____
_____

DIET:_____
_____
_____

TUESDAY

CARDIO:_____
_____
_____

STRENGTH:_____
_____
_____

STRETCHING:_____
_____
_____

DIET:_____
_____
_____

WEDNESDAY

CARDIO:_____
_____
_____

STRENGTH:_____
_____
_____

STRETCHING:_____
_____
_____

DIET:_____
_____
_____
_____

THURSDAY

CARDIO:_____
_____
_____

STRENGTH:_____
_____
_____

STRETCHING:_____
_____
_____

DIET:_____
_____
_____

FRIDAY

CARDIO:_____
_____
_____

STRENGTH:_____
_____
_____

STRETCHING:_____
_____
_____

DIET:_____
_____
_____

SATURDAY

CARDIO:_____
_____
_____

STRENGTH:_____
_____
_____

STRETCHING:_____
_____
_____

DIET:_____
_____
_____

SUNDAY

CARDIO:_____
_____
_____

STRENGTH:_____
_____
_____

STRETCHING:_____
_____
_____

DIET:_____
_____
_____

WEEKLY NOTES:
_____
_____
_____
_____
_____
_____

"The mind is the most important part of achieving any fitness goal. Mental change always comes before physical change." – Matt McGorry

WEEK FIFTY TWO: _____

MONDAY

CARDIO:_____
_____
_____

STRENGTH:_____
_____
_____

STRETCHING:_____
_____
_____

DIET:_____
_____
_____

TUESDAY

CARDIO:_____
_____
_____

STRENGTH:_____
_____
_____

STRETCHING:_____
_____
_____

DIET:_____
_____
_____

WEDNESDAY

CARDIO:_____
_____
_____

STRENGTH:_____
_____
_____

STRETCHING:_____

_____

_____

DIET:_____

_____

_____

_____

THURSDAY

CARDIO:_____

_____

_____

STRENGTH:_____

_____

_____

STRETCHING:_____

_____

_____

DIET:_____

_____

_____

FRIDAY

CARDIO:_____

_____

_____

STRENGTH:_____

_____

_____

STRETCHING:_____

_____

_____

DIET:_____

_____

_____

SATURDAY

CARDIO:_____
_____
_____

STRENGTH:_____
_____
_____

STRETCHING:_____
_____
_____

DIET:_____
_____
_____

SUNDAY

CARDIO:_____
_____
_____

STRENGTH:_____
_____
_____

STRETCHING:_____
_____
_____

DIET:_____
_____
_____

WEEKLY NOTES:
_____
_____
_____
_____
_____
_____
_____

"Fitness is not about being better than someone else … it's about being better than you used to be." – Khloe Kardashian

In Conclusion

There journalling pages in this diary cover a whole year's worth of your exercise and diet regime. However exercise and diet should be a lifetime pastime so feel free to print off as many pages as you want to continue keeping a diary account of your healthy lifestyle.

Below is a handy chart to help you record your healthy lifestyle progress at the end of every 4 weeks, over the 52 weeks that this diary covers. Once again you can print this off so that you can continue to record your progress for as long as you want.

Start of Week One _____

Weight: _____

Measurements
Upper Arm: _____   **Chest/Bust:** _____
Waist: _____   **Hips:** _____
Thighs: _____   **Calves:** _____

Total Workout Minutes
Cardio: _____   **Strength:** _____

End of Week Four _____

Weight: _____

Measurements
Upper Arm: _____   **Chest/Bust:** _____
Waist: _____   **Hips:** _____
Thighs: _____   **Calves:** _____

Total Workout Minutes
Cardio: _____   **Strength:** _____

End of Week Eight _____

Weight: _____

Measurements
Upper Arm: _____   **Chest/Bust:** _____
Waist: _____   **Hips:** _____
Thighs: _____   **Calves:** _____

Total Workout Minutes
Cardio: _____   **Strength:** _____

End of Week Twelve _____

Weight: _____

Measurements
Upper Arm: _____	**Chest/Bust:** _____
Waist: _____	**Hips:** _____
Thighs: _____	**Calves:** _____

Total Workout Minutes
Cardio: _____	**Strength:** _____

End of Week Sixteen _____

Weight: _____

Measurements
Upper Arm: _____	**Chest/Bust:** _____
Waist: _____	**Hips:** _____
Thighs: _____	**Calves:** _____

Total Workout Minutes
Cardio: _____	**Strength:** _____

End of Week Twenty _____

Weight: _____

Measurements
Upper Arm: _____	**Chest/Bust:** _____
Waist: _____	**Hips:** _____
Thighs: _____	**Calves:** _____

Total Workout Minutes
Cardio: _____	**Strength:** _____

End of Week Twenty Four _____

Weight: _____

Measurements
Upper Arm: _____	**Chest/Bust:** _____
Waist: _____	**Hips:** _____
Thighs: _____	**Calves:** _____

Total Workout Minutes
Cardio: _____	**Strength:** _____

End of Week Twenty Eight _____

Weight: _____

Measurements
Upper Arm: _____   **Chest/Bust:** _____
Waist: _____   **Hips:** _____
Thighs: _____   **Calves:** _____

Total Workout Minutes
Cardio: _____   **Strength:** _____

End of Week Thirty Two _____

Weight: _____

Measurements
Upper Arm: _____   **Chest/Bust:** _____
Waist: _____   **Hips:** _____
Thighs: _____   **Calves:** _____

Total Workout Minutes
Cardio: _____   **Strength:** _____

End of Week Thirty Six _____

Weight: _____

Measurements
Upper Arm: _____   **Chest/Bust:** _____
Waist: _____   **Hips:** _____
Thighs: _____   **Calves:** _____

Total Workout Minutes
Cardio: _____   **Strength:** _____

End of Week Forty _____

Weight: _____

Measurements
Upper Arm: _____   **Chest/Bust:** _____
Waist: _____   **Hips:** _____
Thighs: _____   **Calves:** _____

Total Workout Minutes
Cardio: _____   **Strength:** _____

End of Week Forty Four _____

Weight: _____

Measurements
Upper Arm: _____   Chest/Bust: _____
Waist: _____   Hips: _____
Thighs: _____   Calves: _____

Total Workout Minutes
Cardio: _____   Strength: _____

End of Week Forty Eight _____

Weight: _____

Measurements
Upper Arm: _____   Chest/Bust: _____
Waist: _____   Hips: _____
Thighs: _____   Calves: _____

Total Workout Minutes
Cardio: _____   Strength: _____

End of Week Fifty Two _____

Weight: _____

Measurements
Upper Arm: _____   Chest/Bust: _____
Waist: _____   Hips: _____
Thighs: _____   Calves: _____

Total Workout Minutes
Cardio: _____   Strength: _____

CELEBRATE because you have made it through a whole year and have transformed your health and your lifestyle for good.

Finally I wish you all the best in your healthy lifestyle journey, whether it be to lose a few pounds so that you can fit those old blue jeans, or you are aiming to run a marathon.

What matters is that you start this journey and make it a lifelong one because the benefits to you, your life, your friends and your family will astound you.

"Your body is your most priceless possession ...
*   so go take care of it!" – Jack Lalanne*

Books by Jennifer Daniels and Women's Health Blast

Your Guide to the Absolutely Best Healthy YouTube Cooking Videos
Your Guide to the Absolutely Best YouTube Ab Workout Videos

Other books by Jennifer Daniels

Health Checks: DIY Health Checks You Can Do At Home
Great Food Great Health
Getting Older Living Younger
Stomach Pain and Your Colon Health
Jennifer Daniels Health Compendium

All of the above books are only available from Amazon's Kindle Store.

Women's Health Blast
Facebook Page
Website

www.ingramcontent.com/pod-product-compliance
Lightning Source LLC
Chambersburg PA
CBHW071357280526
45787CB00001B/361